Gastric Band
Hypnosis Sessions

George Bren

trademarks and brands within this book are for clarifying purposes only and are the owned by the owners themselves, not affiliated with this document.

INTRODUCTION

This book will elaborate on all these subconscious underlying determinants of weight struggles and how gastric band hypnotherapy can put an end to the misery once and for all.

Gastric band hypnotherapy helps to reveal these underlying causes, helping individuals to eventually push down walls, which could have stopped them from losing weight for so many years. If you are struggling with mindless and emotional eating, gastric band hypnotherapy could help you regain control. The aim is to make you stay fuller for longer, which will assist in avoiding excessive grazing all day long. It is a successful way of confronting your counterproductive attitudes and beliefs in times of distress, enabling you to pursue a healthier lifestyle.

Gastric band hypnotherapy aims to make you more comfortable in your skin, shift unhealthy food beliefs and help you lose weight effectively without disrupting your mental well-being. By incorporating strong hypnotic suggestions to reach the unconscious mind, a hypnotherapist may help you build a productive relationship with healthy eating and exercise, which is essential to safe weight loss and long-term weight control.

So, if you're actually ready and determined to lose weight once and for all and commit both time and money to achieve results, this book is just for you. Before you start your journey, remember that you must desire the change only for your own good and no one else, not the family, not the followers and not the society.

Chapter 1: Gastric Band Hypnosis Sessions

The program entails three to four one-on-one hypnotherapy sessions typically held every week over four weeks. The first session is to be an actual free meeting. This phase in the plan would include a conversation of the dietary patterns, what strategies of weight management have also been tested, emotional health and dietary attitude.

This consultation is a way to gain details about you and ensure that the care is individually customized and fit the preferences better. The practitioner would, therefore, be able to decide whether you are a good candidate for the hypnotherapy treatment or not.

During the actual 'procedure' gastric band, the person is politely directed into hypnosis. This quickly and quite conveniently happens to a stage of deep relaxation, where we can reach their unconscious and increase the sensitivity of the individual to constructive suggestions.

Then, through the process step by step, the therapist guides the person qualitatively through being positioned under general anesthetic and the ride on a stretcher to the operating room. Of course, you feel completely relaxed and safe because there is no pain or irritation whatsoever.

While the patient in hypnotherapy is mindful of what is unfolding around them, because the subconscious mind in hypnosis cannot recognize the distinction between true and imaginary, the lines between what is true and imaginary are blurred, such that interpreting the surgical process under hypnosis will potentially affect the specific emotional reactions the client experiences after the treatment is finished.

Everyone encounters varying results from gastric band hypnotherapy, with certain individuals feeling the sense of actual squeezing of their stomach, whilst some are unable to establish any deliberate link to the 'surgery', but feed less normally and get content with much smaller quantities.

The intention of the operation itself is to imitate that of the actual surgical process, using sound to render the feeling more realistic. You will be brought into a profoundly relaxing condition that will have your heart rate falling to a point not far below the stage at which it falls when you sleep. Then your unconscious can be reached in this condition of intense relaxation, and you'll be much more open to constructive advice.

You would then be guided phase by phase into the process and during the treatment, and while you may be completely calm, you will always be conscious of what is unfolding outside you. You can be brought right under the anesthesia, through the first cut, through the shutting off of the gastric band and placing the last stitch in through the whole process.

What are the causes of failure?

As good and effective as the gastric hypnotic band might be, the plan inevitably isn't going to work for everyone. This is because weight reduction for most people is more about determination and mentality than just calories. Now, this doesn't mean that consuming the right food isn't necessary for weight reduction, but this isn't where people are stumbling and falling.

So, if you find yourself having the problems mentioned below, then odds are not only that the hypnosis treatment of the gastric band would not succeed for you, but no weight reduction method would allow you to be effective and achieve your objectives.

1. You're seeking a magic wand

Hypnosis isn't a mystical cure for overcoming all the problems. Hypnotherapists can't help you perform something you don't want to do, like weight reduction. If you're trying to sign up to the plan and anticipate all the training to be performed by the hypnotherapist, so you lose weight without taking part, then you're wasting time and resources. There is no part of the treatment involving extracting your brain and scrubbing it from the triggers which make you overweight.

2. You expect to fail

A lot of people give latent signals to their subconscious mind that they anticipate struggling at weight loss. One example is those that carry their overweight dresses or suits around only in case they don't succeed, so they get all their weight back.

Others have attempted all the food and fitness regimes at least once and struggled, and so with equal hopes, they join the Virtual Gastric Band hypnosis plan. Their self-talk would be along the lines of "I have really nothing to lose, so I'm going to try it out".

3. You always blame someone else

If you still see yourself finding a reason not to lose weight and blaming someone for failing to succeed in past efforts, then you will have a hard time keeping to the guidelines and dedication needed as part of the plan. It's common that the programmer's first few weeks are nice and relatively easy to follow, but then some obstacles arise, and things get a little harder and then there's a series of excuses to explain why you've "fallen off the road" this week. Detours arise from time to time, and this is fine, but getting constantly interrupted usually implies that there is a problem of commitment that needs to be taken care of.

Hypnosis is a totally natural state of complete relaxation and deep mental concentration that will help you redefine old food habits and values to retain a healthier weight. Using hypnosis, discover the stressful condition that contributed to a defensive reaction arising. Obesity is not just gaining pounds, after all. From the unconscious's point of view, it's your protective shell. A big individual would not be starving to death; obesity is a source of calories in the event of food shortage. A large individual is shielded better from foreign danger. Very commonly, the explanation for accumulating extra weight is actually anxiety. Rewiring your subconscious mind for new behavior with the guidance of hypnosis will just address the issue in tandem with a balanced lifestyle and self-discipline.

As many of you know, gastric band surgery can be very costly and has many risks afterward. This hypnosis session is for adults exclusively over 18 years of age. This is intended to convince your subconscious with the power of hypnosis that a physical gastric band is now put in place. This will help you overcome challenges like unhealthy eating; it will undo negative programming from years of yo-

yo dieting and improve body-image. It will help you with emotional eating, motivation for exercise and learning to love healthy foods. Remember, you're always in control, and you choose to go under hypnosis. You may or may not recall everything suggested to you. But you still choose the suggestions voluntarily; you won't accept suggestions that you're not ready to believe in or those that clash with your goals. So, let's begin.

Session 1 (installing)

Induction

- Find a comfortable place, preferably at home or a quiet room where you won't be disturbed.

- Settle into a chair or bed and close your eyes. As you settle in and relax, take a nice deep inhale, making yourself calm and exhale it very slowly now, releasing tension from the body. Now inhale again and exhale deeply again. Make any adjustments you like. As you do, start to notice your body as you continue taking nice, deep breaths.

- Ensure that your neck and head are supported, as you will get relaxed during this. Let your shoulder and spine loose, and you may wish to let go completely. Feel your back and readjust it, so it is in full contact with the bed or chair you're on. You want to feel completely comfortable. The more comfortable you are, the more profoundly you'll go into hypnosis and the more powerful the effect.

- Feel your breath as you allow your chest to open a little, feeling your shoulders roll back and down. Allow the breath flow more freely. Sitting or lying, legs crossed or straight, and arms crossed or by the side, just connect to your breath now.

- There is no need for absolute stillness; this is not like meditation. If you feel the need to move or adjust, just know that any of these movements will relax you even more. And even if the conscious mind is chattering, your subconscious mind is listening. Know that the mind will stop its chatter and narrow its focus more and more as you continue to follow my voice.

- Now, as you start to scan your body from head to toe like it's a medical scan, except it's a mental scan for relaxation. Beginning at the head, scan your body for where it needs to relax more. Feel at the forehead; let any tension release. Letting go and moving down to scanning your face, relaxing the cheeks, the lips, and the mouth. Deep inhale and releasing the exhale. Loosen the jaw, relax the chin. Let go of any tightness. Down to the neck, scanning all around the neck. Muscles are loosening, noticing your breathing gets easier. Moving down to your shoulders, letting them go now as you sink down deeper. Scan down every vertebra, everything loosens, sink deeper down into the bed or chair. Scan your upper back, middle and lower back. If there is any tension there, release that tension as you settle down. Breathe it out now, and your hips follow, scanning releasing that tension. And scanning the front of your body now, chest already open, and opening up even more now and relaxing even more now as you settle into this safe space. Your tummy relaxes, feeling your stomach now connecting to your body through your throat. Connect to your body and breathe. As your breathe flows down, you notice and feel your body even more as you follow my voice. You're feeling your legs rest, your toes loosening.

The procedure

- As you're welcomed into the room, it feels right you feel so good. You see the equipment, and all concerns melt away now. And now on the bed, you look down, and you're in a medical gown. You feel the anesthetic taking its effect, feeling safe, happy and relaxed, knowing that you'll wake up with everything different in a positive way. This is the start of remarkable changes. You are hearing the distant voices of the surgeon and nurses.

- As they start to prepare, your eyes are getting heavy and eventually close in this scene, and you're aware of observing this scene as if watching and hearing yourself down a tunnel. As you see tiny incisions in your chest, tiny points, smaller than a baby's fingernails. You feel nothing, you know it's happening, but you're safe and protected. The surgeons are talking with each other; they look competent and in control. They know what they're doing. The heart monitor is beeping, and all your vital signs are very good. And you see your chest rise and fall; you see the white of the walls and the blue of the surgeon's scrubs. You see the regular beats of the heart monitor. And you're aware that a small tube goes on through the incision, just a small tube. Here it is now; you see a surgeon using a tube going into the reservoir, and he's placing an inflatable silicone band around the upper part of your stomach. Everyone is silent now, focusing. You feel something at some level touching your stomach, just a touch. All is good, and the surgeon starts to adjust this. And as you observe yourself, you feel this coming into place, wrapping the band around the upper part of your stomach. You feel it; it is just a slight touch. Creating a small pouch with the band, you feel the squeeze just a little.

- As you are so connected to your body right now, you start to feel the difference. And now, the surgeon is adjusting the band. It is just like a small belt around your stomach, squeezing the stomach in to create that pouch. And you know food ad digestion still flows normally, and as they adjust it, you feel so good already. This has already been so much easier than you thought, and you feel a difference already. You already know you'll eat differently from now on, from this day on. You notice a different sensation around your stomach, and you feel good.

- As they make final adjustments and start to complete the procedure, placing a few stitches and your vital signs are good and regular. The last stitch is in place; everything is clean and well done. The surgeons are all calm and happy with a job well done. They check that you are fine and then allow you to come back up as the anesthetic starts to wear off. You're still staying down just relaxing. And sometime after, you see yourself fully healed, feeling the band in place. And you know that every time you eat now when you wake up, you not only eat less but you spend more time eating, slowing down as you get fuller faster from this day on. You promise to enjoy every mouthful, every bite, and every snack. When you wake up, you no longer eat till you're stuffed. Instead, you naturally adjust your scale of appetite. You know that you eat just enough, never too much. As your stomach is smaller, your portion size is smaller. You hour your body. You now eat intuitively. You notice your stomach is already flatter and have more energy. You feel so proud. Just take one last look at the future you. You're getting up slowly with 6…letting the last grogginess out of your body and 7…feeling a tingling in your toes and 8…moving your body a little and 9…committing to that image of slimmer you and 10…you wake up with eyes open as you exhale.

Session 2 (tightening)

Use the previously mentioned induction method before gastric band tightening hypnosis.

- As you lie down completely relaxed, you can hear the surgeon preparing the saline injection to tighten your gastric band. Feel the air, sound and smell in the room. You're feeling very calm.

- You are observing yourself from the outside. Now you are hearing the surgeon wear his gloves to do the short procedure. Relax and breathe deeply. The skin around your reservoir is being cleaned now. Feel the alcohol swab cooling your skin. Now the surgeon is gently removing the swab. You're now feeling his hands on your stomach as he tries to feel the soft part of the gastric band port to inject saline. You're calm and relaxed. Breathe in and out deeply. Now the surgeon is injecting the saline solution into your gastric band. As the saline slowly moves through the tube and towards the band, you can feel a slight tightening in your stomach. You're feeling that your stomach has shrunken even further. It feels like your stomach pouch is getting smaller and smaller. It's all very comfortable, and you feel at ease. Everything is going well.

- Now the surgeon is finishing up the procedure. You can hear the nurse congratulating the surgeon on successful tightening. Everything is going smooth and clean, and you feel absolutely amazing. You're feeling a bandage being placed on the injection site. And you feel calm and happy as you get up slowly.

Session 3 (removal)

Use the previously mentioned induction method before gastric band removal hypnosis.

- As you look down, you're wearing a hospital gown, and the surgeons and nurses around you are preparing for the procedure. You are completely relaxed, lying down on your back. The room temperature is very comfortably cool. You are hearing the doctors and nurses chat about how the gastric band will be removed. You're observing yourself from the outside. You're feeling the inhaled anesthesia in your nose. It is kicking in slowly, and you start to feel sleepy. Your eyes are feeling heavy.

- As you breathe in, feel the surgeon re-opening the tiny incisions made during the installation procedure. You feel extremely at ease and relaxed as the surgeon cuts the scar tissue around the band. Then, he cuts the tubing attached and the gastric band itself. You now feel a relief in your stomach. Feel the doctor pulling out the gastric band from around your stomach. You are at total peace now. You can feel it all just like a slight touch. You see your ideal self that you've always wanted to be, and you have become that now.

- Now, the doctor is removing the sutures on your stomach. You are very relaxed now. Hear the heart rate monitor beeping regularly. See the operation theater bulbs over your head. The subcutaneous band reservoir is getting removed now. The incisions are now being stitched up.

- The procedure is complete. You feel the anesthesia wearing off now. The surgeons are really happy with the job well done. You are slowly waking up now in 3, 2, and 1.

Chapter 2: Overcome Food Addiction with Hypnosis

There is really nothing that can make or break your weight loss efforts completely, as mindful eating does. When you can't control your emotions, and they run the show for you, you fall into the trap of food addiction. But there is a way out, i.e., gastric band hypnotherapy. This procedure is perfect for people who have long struggled with emotional eating for decades. In this chapter, we'll talk about mindful and mindless eating, what causes mindless eating, how it hampers weight loss and what you can do about it

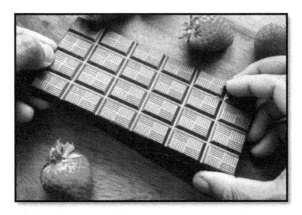

2.1 What is mindful eating?

Mindful eating is based on the Buddhist principle of mindfulness. Mindful eating is a strategy that lets you take mastery of eating patterns. It has been shown that it encourages weight reduction, decreases binge eating and makes you experience better health. To feed consciously is not really a diet. It uses a method of meditation called mindfulness, which lets you identify and control your bodily experiences and emotions. Using this method will help you enter a state of total understanding of your food habits, cravings and physical signals.

The goal of mindful eating is to help yourself to be conscious of the meaningful and rewarding opportunities available by selection and food preparation through embracing your true self. It also involves utilizing all your sensations in deciding to consume food that stimulates you as well as nourishes your body. As well as accepting reactions to food (like hate or unbiased) without judgment, you become mindful of physical appetite and satiety signs to direct your eating preferences to begin and finish.

Mindful eating entails:

- Understanding that no right or incorrect form of eating exists

- There is a variety of understanding of the dietary patterns

- To acknowledge that eating habits are different for everyone

- Turning your focus to feeding moment by moment

- Understanding how you create fitness and wellness decisions

- To become conscious of the Earth's interconnection with living things and cultural traditions and the effect of your decisions on them.

- Cultivating harmony, preference, insight and acceptability

Mindless eating

Do you find yourself shocked by the number of cookies, sweets you consumed at a briefing? Yeah, that's known as mindless eating. Mindless feeding involves consuming without stimulating the brain. It's a type of eating amnesia; you place snacks in your mouth without paying close attention to what is actually being consumed mindlessly, and how much. You can talk, compose or view the TV as you feed. In this scenario, it is eating meals in a meeting or conference.

It is really easy to slip into unhealthy eating while you are at a conference. The food (might) is there, right in front of you, and you're not engaged too vigorously in operation.

It is dangerous to feed thoughtlessly. It contributes to bad food choices, which aggravate your attempts to maintain your diet and lifestyle. And when you consume, you are not full, the sugar spike in you rises, you end up consuming more, and gradually gaining weight.

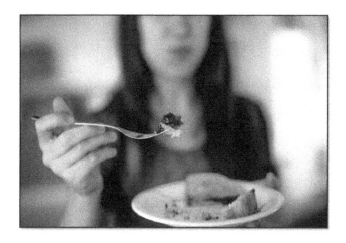

2.2 Causes of mindless eating

There are many explanations for why someone could consume without knowing how much they do. Eating when we're sad may bring us relief, especially foods that we really love (usually sugary snacks). 'Treating ourselves to a delicious breakfast or pie is normal because while we're stressed out, plenty of us want to settle down in front of the Television with our favorite tasty treat and relax. Tiredness is also a major source of mindless feeding because while we feed and do something else, for example, watching a film or sitting at our offices, we are more apt to consume than we should.

1. Eating meals at fixed times

You could be consuming your meals at fixed hours, the manner your life is organized. Perhaps your work needs you to take your lunch hour in the afternoon every day. Or, every evening, you sit and eat alongside your parents at a fixed time. Eating at fixed hours is normal for people, particularly though they are not feeling hungry. One effective route to deal with this is to ask yourself if you are still hungry as you sit down at each dinner. To stop food once you are indeed full, it is super healthy for the body and for weight loss purposes.

2. Eating when doing something else

For several people, one of the popular behaviors is to feed when doing something different. Any evening you may eat dinner at the front of the Screen. Or, you may eat your dinner while you browse the net. It is yet another indication that excessive feeding happens as part of social interaction. You might not be tuning into whether or not you're bingeing or whether you're chewing your food properly while your focus is on another task.

3. Eating to kill time

Another indication of unhealthy feeding is eating while bored. This can happen individually or when you call a mate, even though you're not hungry, to go outside for dinner or a snack. Any meal you eat when you're not starving is an emotional illustration. In these situations, food satisfies a function apart from feeding the appetite and supplying calories.

4. Sounds, sights, and smells

Just the seductive scent of bacon cooking, or the sight

of kernels popping, will cause overeating, or just passing by the baker display with all of those freshly made chocolate chip cookies on sale.

5. Huge portions

Our definition of a reasonable portion has been warped, partially because there are too many places offering large portions. Cautious eating will also benefit here. Eat gently, put the spoon down in between bites, sample the food and be more in tune with what you consume and how it feels, so you can love it more and begin appreciating pleasure for smaller amounts of it.

6. Fear of starvation

You may have heard of this phrase, "Take some bread or you might starve to death!" Fear of eventual hunger is a reason to feed a number of people. Malnutrition is the toughest thing imaginable, and hunger may be a terrifying sensation for certain people with a history of dieting! The fear about not seeing a single meal again – you're on a family break and not sure when you're going to get the ability to have the meal again, but you're starving, and you don't want to hurt yourself. Another consideration is the fear of missing out on the meal. You're not hungry, but there's food in the fridge, and you don't want anyone to have it before you do, so you'll enjoy it!

2.3 Emotional eating – a barrier to weight loss

Emotional eating corresponds to food intake with the intention of controlling one's emotional processes. Eating palatable foods usually candy, salty, or foods high in carbs can momentarily boost our mood, but that short-lived relief comes at the risk of excess weight and other health concerns.

You may have been programmed to eat over time when you're feeling unhappy, upset, stressed or injured. It is not important to investigate the specific historical explanation for this, so when you were unhappy as a kid, it might have been related to a circumstance of stimulation/response such as food being provided. You might have begun to see food as a relief as a whole anything to 'take away the discomfort'. You may have used sugar as a distraction from other problems of your life; it helps you feel easier when you're enjoying it, so when you sit to consider how much you've consumed, you feel bad-now you're consuming more to feel comfortable again. It is a twisted cycle of nightmares. You will also search for the brief 'rush' that arises from sugar drinks, which can raise your blood glucose levels and help you feel great, but also, your blood glucose levels can drop really easily and make you feel much worse afterward.

Our minds are programmed to sustain an endorphin level, which makes us feel healthy. As these amounts are low due to tension or distress, we always need something to give us a 'fix' (basically something to raise our endorphin levels). A very easy way to achieve this is to consume something sweet or sugar-so we recognize, of course, it's not good for us because we get a brief relief from the negative feelings inside, so we realize we're doing ourselves damage in the long run-and that makes us feel terrible again.

Over the span of many years, each of us accepts our own particular encounters through which food has given a form of both emotional and physical security. You could have been offered a bottle as an infant, for example, because you were upset, no matter why you were sobbing. The baby's mind sends out the idea that people give me something to make me feel better when I'm unhappy or frustrated or tired or lonely. When you were a child, ice-cream was possibly combined with fun occasions or holidays, as well as being "good" or playing a "great game". there are about as many instances as people are. Your "Comfort Food Chart" is different from others.

Dietary phases, reducing calorie consumption and

switching between phases of bingeing and abusing the normal appetite rhythms of the body can mess with the indicators of the internal appetite. You could have gone without experiencing real hunger for years because you're too busy satisfying your mental appetite to encourage you to be hungry physically. Or else you hungered yourself on diets and didn't satisfy your actual appetite-having your body believe it was starved of food, and therefore holding it on calories (energy) by storing fat-making you overweight. And you only have to teach yourself to feed while you're mentally starving.

We'll let you in on a bit of a secret: we're all emotional eaters. We bring the food to relatives and friends, to display our care and interest, we make our kids their favorite meals to demonstrate our affection for them, we share pleasant times with a fancy meal, we offer our babe chocolates as an affirmation of our affection, and we prefer meals like mac n' cheese, or a fluffy pot-pie, anytime we want a warm and relaxing experience.

When we're concerned about emotional eating these days, it's because we've been physically reliant on unhealthy behaviors such as binge eating, excessive dieting, body-hating, pessimistic self-talk, and compulsive overeating. Or when we misuse food as our main means to deal with and control our emotions. But the solution to these questions is not to shut ourselves off from emotion, but rather to suggest the need for a more positive and caring food partnership to improve our overall health.

Subconscious and food choices

There was no other huge amount of food here at any point. Being well-balanced and stable should be easy. In reality, ever more individuals are becoming fat, and illnesses linked to obesity are becoming common. How would it fit in? Our brain "drives" on auto mode, which is the subconscious, as already described, 95 percent of the time. For example, our brain needs to make thousands of choices every day, on which leg we get out of our bed, how we decide to brush our teeth, and so on. We don't care about those choices at all, since they happen instinctively.

Our subconscious requires much fewer resources than our rational awareness, which is healthier for our bodies. That's why it wants to work as frequently as possible on auto mode (subconscious) and consume fewer resources.

Food options also run on autopilot. This is also relevant to our dietary habits throughout our regular lives. We browse, prepare and consume solely on autopilot much of the time. This automatic method of decision-making is founded on intuition and instinct. We eat the way we are accustomed to. The unconscious aspect stems from the origins of mankind, which we wanted back then to live. That implies, as we determine subconsciously what to consume, our instincts advise us to take really quickly whatever food provides tons of calories.

That's just what we wanted to live back then since we didn't know when we'd have access to resources next time.

The same holds valid with our patterns; they always deceive us into making food decisions that aren't good for us. When we're on auto mode and remember that we're hungry in the evening, chocolate could come to our mind right away. It's nice; we've always enjoyed it as a child, it's accessible almost anywhere, and we can consume it quickly. Of course, instincts and routines aren't a negative thing; we need them to function. We sure don't want to intentionally make every single choice. That means the day will be done, and we'd hardly make it from bed to bathroom.

As you all know by now, emotional eating is one of the biggest factors responsible for your weight gain. You are consuming food as a way to suppress your negative emotion such as anger, stress, boredom, loneliness and sadness. Hypnosis can help you rectify this particular problem.

The best advice is combining a healthy meal plan and exercise with hypnosis. If you manage to follow along with this routine, you definitely can reach and maintain your ideal body weight goal.

2.4 Tips to overcome emotional eating

 Changing our subconscious is not straightforward. To alter it, we need to be more aware. This implies, precisely, that we need to do what our mind and body are attempting to escape. We have to learn to shift from autopilot to consciousness to use willpower to create more decisions than normal. At some stage, we have rewired our unconscious to take a different path instinctively, for instance, rather than picking chocolate, picking an apple automatically.

We need to stop the automatism and question ourselves if I really do want to consume this right away or if there are any other available options?

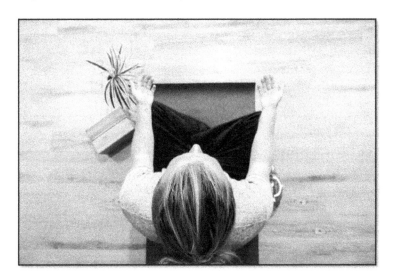

1. Keep a food and mood journal

For those of us, food is a replacement for our emotional needs. If we can understand our desires, write them down, show them plainly on a screen and affirm them as legitimate – so we have a greater chance at discovering solutions to fulfill our desires rather than having food as a supplement to satisfy them.

2. Keep a need and wants list

An effective tool for emotional eating is making a checklist of what we really need, what we want and what we wish for. For certain of us, a diet will satisfy our unmet needs. If we can understand our desires, write them down, show them plainly on a document and affirm them as legitimate – so we have a greater chance of discovering solutions to satisfy our desires, rather than having food as a tool for meeting our yearnings.

3. Serve your food front and center

It's not just simpler to over-eat because you can't tell how many you've eaten, but it's even tougher to completely enjoy your meal because it's concealed from the display.

4. Choose a smaller plate

If you see fewer, you may want fewer. Smaller plates

can aid improve the portion control a very effective tactic for those all-you-can-eat dine outs. If you see fewer, you may want fewer. Smaller plates can aid improve the portion control a very effective tactic for all those all-you-can-eat buffets.

5. Give gratitude

Before you start feeding, stop and take a moment to consider the effort that went into delivering your meal whether it was gratitude to the producers, the factory employees, the poultry, mother nature, the chef or even your fellows at the table.

Try to consume your meals in solitude every now and then. While it's silent, it's normal for the mind to roam; accept these feelings and then see how you can subtly switch back to your eating experience. Be mindful of the consistency, color, texture and scent of the food and thoroughly enjoy the moment.

6. Chew your food 30 times

Try having 30 chews out of a slice. (30 is a tough plan,

so it may be challenging to take even ten chews out of a spoonful of granola!). Take some time to savor the tastes and textures of your mouth before swallowing. This will also benefit by allowing your stomach time to transmit signals to the brain that tell you're full.

7. Leave the *clean plate* team

All of us were brought up to finish all on our plate and had not been permitted to quit the table before we did. Canceling your affiliation at Clean Plate Team is perfect. Try throwing away the leftover food, or maybe save the remaining few bites. While no one enjoys wasting calories, over-stuffing oneself would not benefit people in need.

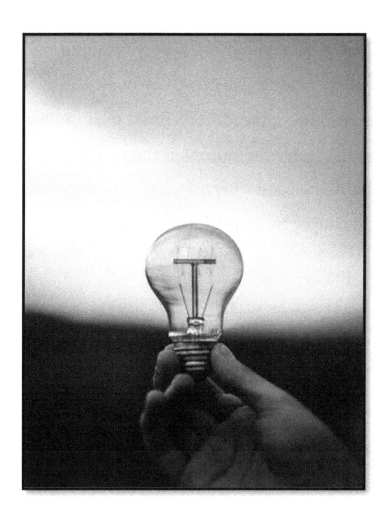

Chapter 3: Change Your Mindset to Lose Weight

Any diet or weight-loss plan has its benefits and drawbacks, so you have to keep your mind right for it to actually work. The greatest weight-loss aspect is changing the mindset on how to lose weight. Without understanding the right inner determination and purpose, we cannot change our weight simply from outside.

Often people want to shed weight in the worst imaginable state of mind, i.e., trying to "repair" themselves. They fall into diets and workout schedules out of self-loathing. It is not only about having a positive mindset and "feeling good" that will allow you to shed weight; it is also about results. Luckily, mindset and beliefs can always be changed with hypnosis. In this chapter of the book, we will elaborate on the importance of limiting beliefs and how much impact they have when it comes to losing weight. We'll also talk about the common limiting beliefs that hinder weight loss, and 2how hypnosis can help you overcome such a mindset. Lastly, we'll mention two exercises to remove your self-sabotaging limiting beliefs.

3.1 How limiting beliefs sabotage weight loss

Even though you know the correct path ahead for you, and you can confidently see what the ideal potential feels like and sounds like, you do have assumptions in yourself that keep you hostage. If you've been counting calories and abusing your body with unhealthy food for years, you may have a very low perception of yourself. You have to suppress the inner voice undermining your ambitions and being counterproductive. If you ever think you don't have what is needed to create improvements that can last a lifetime and end in a fresh, lean, balanced you, now is the time to make changes.

Patients of weight loss sometimes display old or generally unhelpful beliefs and experiences, some from infancy, some acquired all along the way as they pass throughout life. Typically, these emerge in one manner or another; also, during the induction period, a person can have information to particular views or feelings that may not correspond to their overall intention to be healthy.

The point is that you may actively want something, but something is in the subconsciousness that prevents you from getting what you want. And until you remove the barrier (limiting belief) in your subconsciousness, weight reduction probably won't happen. This one truth in our subconscious is buried deep inside. And unlike your waking mind, you must understand that your subconscious mind never rests.

Everything you do during the waking moments, you store certain interactions and the responses to them in brain cells. This section of the brain functions like a machine that records everything you've heard since your infancy or witnessed.

The first seven years of our existence are also critical. It is the most meaningful time of our existence. A child's very first six years of life are lived in an entrancing condition. Everything occurs, everything that is observed at that moment, all acquired patterns, all are transferred directly into our subconscious.

This implicit conditioning is imported by gazing at the actions of someone. Any time anyone suggests that you are not nice enough, or that you are not lovable, or that you are not clever enough, or that you deserve nothing. Much of it turns into a part of shaping our subconscious. And you, most of the time, work on flawed internal programming! We often develop restricting assumptions as we replicate a concept over and over. And if you're constantly worrying: "It's very difficult to lose weight. It really is difficult. It's so hard". Then, it would become a conviction preventing you from within.

The number one explanation people fail is that they refuse to make adjustments to their inner minds in order to achieve their active objectives. They're let down by their subconscious mind by pushing them down. We become captives of our "present programming" in a way. That's something that occurs to some extent to everybody, part upbringing, part shaping of our behaviors, and part protective mechanism. For instance, whether you're overweight, you're likely to have been for too long or dealing with reducing weight all your life, you have well-established habits of over-thinking regarding food, exercise behavior patterns, values, likes, and dislikes regarding diet and exercise that you're both comfortable with and are usual to you.

Common limiting belief about weight loss

It may be challenging to shake these psychological habits and adjust the cognitive functions. On a deeper level, you've grown too used to the existing habits of conduct, the subconscious mind rejects any adjustments when you go beyond everything it understands, and to defend you, it does this. A major shift in your life leaves you naked, helpless and open to more loss; if it can regress you back to your usual ways of thought and actions (which it sees as productive and normal), then it is guarding you.

1. I simply can't do it

If you've tried to lose weight any number of times before, without results, you might find yourself dealing with a deep conviction that you can't lose weight. You may assume you can just lose too much weight, or you might think you can't lose much at all. Anyway, the urge to eat well and workout can overcome this kind of conviction because it feels like a relentless fight to keep moving and make some change at all.

2. I don't even deserve this

Low self-esteem will make you feel like a loser, particularly though you are attempting to make the right steps towards a healthier body weight. If you frequently feel like you don't deserve to have a slim, beautiful body, be sure to begin improving your self-esteem by stating every day, "I deserve to have a good, safe life, and the acts I take today will make this work for me".

3. My family has always been overweight

You may recognize at some level that just because your parents are overweight doesn't imply you must be too, but you might feel as though your genes function against you. The trouble with this idea is that you won't feel confident enough to attempt and reduce weight; you'll only think you'll stay heavy too since all of your relatives are big. To resolve this misconception, note that there are lots of obese households with one or multiple people not dealing with obesity. Know though that Behaviors are passed on through families more frequently than not, and these patterns lead far more to obesity concerns than chromosomes do.

4. I will become vulnerable

Some individuals don't know that they're not heavy simply because of dietary patterns. More frequently than not, as a defensive strategy, there are many internal pressures and traumatic experiences that trigger them to pile on the pounds. With the additional weight on their bodies, they feel better or more secure because, as they start losing weight, they wind up feeling really insecure because they feel exposed. If this is also the case for you, keep aware that excess weight does not always shield you from something. If anything, it complicates your life, psychologically, emotionally and mentally! Be ready to let go of your weight to feel more flexible, and you'll hopefully find a deep reservoir of power that you didn't even realize you've got.

Some of the other limiting beliefs include:

- "My bones just seem to be too wide"

- "Better be big and grateful, than big and sad"

- "Obviously, some people are slim, and some are not so slim"

- "We all are unable to keep in shape after a certain age"

- "The best way to scale back is to suffer from starvation"

- "When I try to lose a few pounds, I actually end up gaining more. So, to even attempt is folly"

- "It takes so long, and I just cannot handle it"

- "Food cannot be tossed out, since kids are hungry in Africa"

- "Carbohydrates make me big"

- "If I get thin, my sister will feel sad, because she's not thin"

- "I've got a sluggish metabolism"

- "Once I lose weight, I cannot keep it off"

- "I risk dropping weight and getting slim because men are going to find me beautiful and take full advantage of me"

- "I was never lean. For me, it really isn't realistic"

- "I'm being robbed of my favorite meals"

4.2 How hypnosis helps to instill weight loss mindset

Hypnosis may play a major role in assisting you in transcending restricting convictions and build new ones. Not all convictions fail instantly. Overcoming the latent reluctance will take some time. The purpose of hypnosis programs, though, is to help an individual eliminate as much of the negative beliefs as necessary entirely and to attempt to reduce the intensity of the others.

By using effective methods in hypnotherapy, a hypnotist will undermine a person's allegiance to his or her convictions and bring in optimistic changes by "implanting" new ideas and promoting a mindset that is more apt to attain a person's goals. Hypnotherapy often helps an individual to understand implicitly how such values can cause issues for them. This strategy is underpinned by the notion that we should reflect less as to whether a conviction is "real" and more on its effect on our lives. When anyone tends to think this way, they will more readily discard unhelpful views.

You open a package that contains popcorn, nachos, potato chips and chocolate. The list is infinite, and the packet is gone before you realize it, and you're left questioning why you consumed too much.

You were not even starving yet! It's really normal for us to wind up consuming out of routine, hunger, or the habit. Some of it is physical, and half is mental. The desire or need to eat is subconscious, so we don't have a real need to consume; we only want "something". If there were really a real requirement, we would be physically hungry.

The other aspect of excessive feeding or munching is that it will cause the release into the brain of those "feel good" chemicals. This produces a subtle feeling of well-being and pleasure that feels more like a benefit we get for feeding. The concern is that it's a short-lived experience and stimulates the need for more. This provides a mechanism of physical and psychological reinforcement that can come into action over and over again.

We may continue to fight, but the minds and bodies start to desire the sense of reward even if only for a brief while, then it becomes an ongoing struggle that more and more individuals wind up failing again.

Hypnosis doesn't really cure weight symptoms but also deals with the reasons for becoming overweight. Hypnosis can also disrupt the loop of gratification and help patients gain mastery over cravings, impulses and over-snacking. Often people feel powerful and positive, particularly when things are going well. They are inspired to achieve their ambitions and feel that they will keep in charge all day long and making healthy eating decisions.

And at work or at home, anytime the smallest problem pops up. The individual who was so optimistic an hour prior suddenly finds himself looking for something they don't really need. Hypnosis may be a huge aid in disrupting this loop of unhealthy eating decisions and bad food choices and diet addictions. Hypnosis focused weight reduction method offers you the diet schedule you need to successfully lose fat. It gives you the self-belief that you can achieve it by yourself. You can push through, and in the long run, you will lose weight.

The unconscious mind's strength is exceptional. Tap into this ability to make the subconscious function in your advantage, instead of sabotaging yourself. It can help you meet your weight reduction targets without a lack of belief. You would see the progress you are about to accomplish in your head, and then render that your current reality. You will exit every session of weight loss hypnosis with restored confidence that you can meet every health and fitness target you have. This inner commitment and self-confidence render eating your new way of life healthier without the willpower involved. You don't need willpower, and the journey of moving to a healthy diet would really satisfy you.

Hypnosis may be the component that the weight-loss efforts have often lacked. Trying to achieve it with diet alone or motivation alone will contribute to dissatisfaction and, due to lack of success, ultimately to leave. Hypnosis therapy would reverse the bad influence of those old derogatory beliefs; however, they started. When you relax and focus, you may find you are soon starting to feel much relaxed and more positive regarding yourself. You should peacefully look at certain old convictions, without being frustrated or disturbed. You tend to feel very disconnected and removed from restricting your beliefs, as though they are actually meaningless to you. You are becoming really excited about what you are going to do about your new rights. You start taking the first actions which can contribute to real-life improvements. You enjoy the idea of freedom.

What you can do

The dilemma at present is that these assumptions work on a subconscious basis. We don't even consider their involvement, far less than they have a significant impact on our actions. Although they are surmounted by several various means, the best thing is to consider their presence in the first place.

Exercise conscious awareness; one of the easiest strategies to overcome our internal barriers to weight reduction is to retain as much consciousness as possible. By actively selecting fresh and more constructive ideas, we will rewire our minds and rewire our bodies to create permanent improvements, instead of thinking, again and again, the same old self-limiting feelings. When we stay in active consciousness, we will strive harder to teach our mind new training rather than going to the same old harmful neural reinforcement loops that we have depended on all of our existence.

Limiting beliefs exercise 1

1. Write down all the negative limiting beliefs about yourself in your journal, e.g., "I won't be able to sustain my weight loss as I still fail at everything in life".

2. Think what your doubting convictions would be like if they were true, and imagine what your existence would seem to be as a result.

3. Now envision what your future would look like if the opposite of your belief was true, for example,

"with the right plan and encouragement, I'm making everything I want a success". Move through this view of your life and consider what the current confidence feels like.

4. Jot down from your experience at least four examples that contradict your restricting beliefs and transform them into something you are very effective at. And question yourself if your self-loathing convictions really are true. Assumptions can evolve over your lifetime; there are several beliefs you used to think you wouldn't recognize as true today (Easter bunny, the Santa clause, your mother had the answer to everything, or all the adults above the age of thirty were outdated). You may think of your old self-limiting beliefs as things you once believed, but you now acknowledge that they are not valid.

Limiting beliefs exercise 2

When you renovate your home, you are searching

for stuff that you want to change; it's no different from renovating your convictions. What healthier belief would you like to swap with an existing one?

- Truly dive straight into what you intend to improve, or what you want to achieve. Your beliefs might be like this. "I believe that anyone food is not "good" or "evil", it is just cause and effect, and I can decide if a food is safe for me or not depending on how I feel after consuming those foods by adjusting my body and following its cues and feedback. This conviction frees you from selecting those things, not by the judgment you place on food, but by how you feel regarding certain foods.

- Then, set a target you'd like to accomplish in regards to diet and lifestyle. So be really straightforward on what you intend to do. Is it losing weight, a clear mindset? Having more energy? Want a more compassionate approach to treat yourself?

- Now, write all your goals down.

- Then, write down what you believe is required to accomplish your target. If your goal is to lose weight, then what do you actually believe is going to carry you there. What do you subconsciously believe needs to happen before you lose weight? Do you eat and value your body instinctively? Are there any particular foods that you wish to minimize? Will that leave you feeling dissatisfied or content with the lifestyle that you create? Render your current convictions fun to you, and true to you.

- Now live your life in harmony with your convictions.

Chapter 5: Positive Self-Talk and Weight Loss

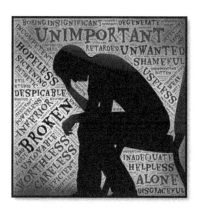

5.1 The significance of positive self-talk

Self-talk is the story inside you that you tell yourself. It is your speech inside, and you may or may not have spent significant time learning about it or paying attention to it. The fact is, our self-talk will potentially affect the way we view ourselves and the environment around us, even more than we know. The most strong self-talk is the implicit monologue you don't really know about, the beliefs and perceptions you've embraced and don't really doubt scripts that will undermine your life and goals. On the other side, if your self-talk is positive, it will drive you towards the paths for which you wish, make your wishes come true and satisfy your lives.

Much of the self-talk we've stumbled through is derogatory, but we didn't know any better. We didn't know how mighty and detrimental this was. An illustration of this is the "I am so huge". Another explanation is, "I still gain weight, no matter what I do", or "I just gain weight by staring at the food".

Self-talk, whether positive or self-destructive, has a somewhat mystical influence, and it contains neurological processes that govern involuntary behavior what you do, automatically think and feel. It programs your subconscious, a strange force capable of controlling your existence.

Positive self-talking is essential for a variety of reasons, as the research indicates. From helping to resolve body dysmorphia to athletic excellence, resolving worry and stress, to learning more effectively: constructive self-talking will create a change for a person.

5.2 Use hypnosis to develop positive self-talk

Our subconscious is like a computer, a system, and the information and programs that it holds and operates are not a question of merely choosing what you would want. Your desktop cannot accomplish what you intend it to do simply by wanting it to, because your robot-like subconscious will not. You have to understand how to configure things, and then you really have to do the rewiring task.

Self-hypnosis and autosuggestion are the ways to how you can reprogram and rewire your subconscious mind. Hypnosis relates to being calm and concentrated, and imagining things, positive or negative, or dreaming. There is a process when a section of the mind acknowledges this order, or idea, and proceeds to work to carry it out. It is something that we have been doing without understanding since day one. If you've been saying, "I gain weight no matter what I do", there's a part of your consciousness going to function on this idea, and it's possible that you'll feel like consuming and lazing about.

To take better advantage of this phenomenon, you must establish self-talk scripts that are self-promoting, removing the old self-defeating scripts. They must be convincing, or they'll be dismissed by the subconscious. Looking into the mirror, for example, and thinking, "I'm so slim" because you're not, won't help, and you'll think, "No, I'm not", which is the same as "I'm so big".

But instead of thinking, "I'm too fat", you're saying, "I realize there's a fit me inside since I'm wearing a huge fat suit, I would like to get rid of. I'm going to burn it away". You're saying", the true me, the way I was built was always fit inside.

I can burn the fat too. I burn off some weight every

day when I eat less. You are writing a new script instead of thinking, "Never mind, whatever I do ends me up in gaining weight".

5.3 Weight loss affirmations

Understand that you are the one in charge by using weight reduction affirmations and emphasis on increasing self-esteem. Every day is a gradual move

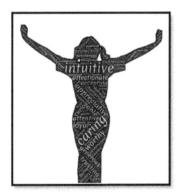

ahead, every time you practice affirmations of encouraging self-talk and weight loss, you reinforce the pathways in your mind, which produce positive outcomes.

1. I have devoted myself to a healthy lifestyle.

2. Before consuming my meal, I honor it.

3. Now I am so thankful for developing good eating habits.

4. I make wise decisions about food.

5. Each day is a fresh start.

6. I love the process of my weight loss. I will finish what I began this time.

7. I consume in the right portions.

8. To me, a good diet comes easily.

9. Exercising naturally appeals to me.

10. I am keeping my focus on my perfect size.

11. I make time to do some workout.

12. My metabolic rate is at its peak and makes me achieve my target weight.

13. I love myself without reservation.

14. Any physical action I do reduces the excess fat in my system and lets me hold my weight at its best.

15. I manage my weight effectively by combining balanced food and exercise.

16. I love to be in this lovely body.

17. I'm enjoying food that brings me energy and leaves me feeling healthy.

18. When I use my muscles, I feel alive and strong.

19. Working out reduces stress and anxiety. The more I exercise, the more relaxed I feel.

20. Food is my energy; I put clean, balanced fuel in my body.

21. I feel comfortable inside this body.

22. I regard this body with love and respect.

23. I love to consume well-balanced food.

24. In my physical endurance and strength, I work out and get the effects straight away.

25. I am strong, fantastic and invincible. I can attain the body I like.

CONCLUSION

A whole chapter was dedicated to introducing the concept of gastric band hypnotherapy. We started off by introducing the idea behind a hypnotic gastric band and its purpose, along with its key benefits and why it is better than an actual surgical gastric band. It is very important to know if the hypnotic gastric band will work for you or not, as it might not. It is considered best for individuals who have at least 25 extra kilograms to lose and those who have struggled with emotional eating for years. On that note, a section was included for the signs that make anyone less eligible for the procedure and might contribute to the failure of the procedure. It includes a lack of discipline, scapegoating others for past failures and looking for a quick fix because there are no quick fixes in life.

Additionally, a whole chapter was dedicated to the most prominent reason behind so many people's weight troubles, i.e., emotional eating. We not only covered the topic of mindful eating but also discussed the causes of mindless eating, which might have been shocking for many of you. This chapter was all about how in times of crisis, our subconscious reverts back to its old familiar ways of soothing itself, i.e., by eating unhealthy but yummy foods. We highlighted the importance of respecting your body's hunger and satiety cues along with tips on how to actually listen to the body and eat mindfully.

The last two chapters covered everything about your mindset and self-talk, which often sabotage your progress and subconsciously force you to act in self-destructive ways. In the end, we elaborated on how gastric band hypnotherapy can be your savior when it comes to a negative self-loathing mental monologue or self-doubting convictions, as it tends to not only put a virtual band on your stomach but also fix the underlying causes and voices that often lead to failure. Finally, a list of daily weight loss affirmations was shared to help you break all your limiting beliefs and rewire you for success.